My Mediterranean Seafood Cookbook

50 Delicious Vegetables & Seafood Mediterranean Recipes

Alex Brawn

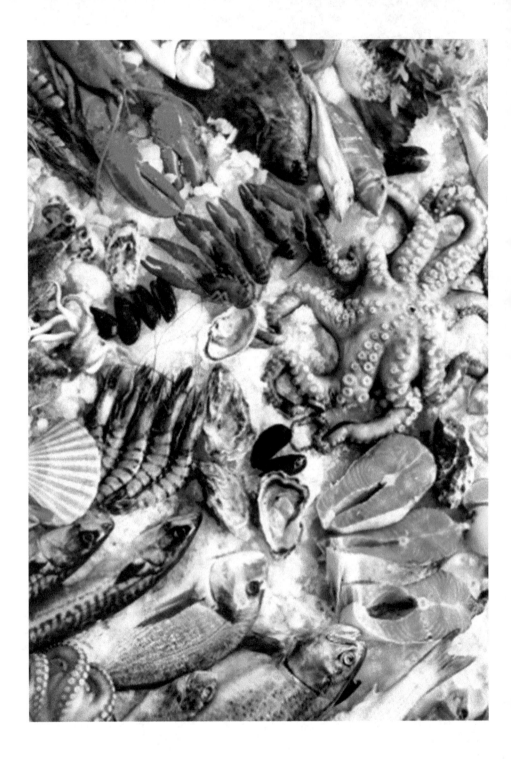

By reading this document, the reader agrees that under no circumstances is the author responsible for any losses, direct or indirect, which are incurred as a result of the use of information contained within this document, including, but not limited to, — errors, omissions, or inaccuracies.

Table of Contents

Hearty sweet potatoes, arugula, and wild rice salad with ginger dressing

Ingredients

- 1 tablespoon of maple syrup or honey
- 1 cup of wild rice, rinsed
- Fine sea salt, divided
- 2 teaspoons of finely grated fresh ginger
- 1 ½ pounds of sweet potatoes
- 2 tablespoons of apple cider vinegar
- Extra virgin olive oil
- ¾ cup of raw pepitas
- 20 twists of freshly ground black pepper
- 2 tablespoons of Dijon mustard
- ¼ cup of dried cranberries
- 5 ounces of arugula
- ½ cup of crumbled feta
- ½ cup of thinly sliced green onion

Directions

- Preheat the oven to 425°F.
- Line a large baking sheet with parchment paper.
- Bring a *large* pot of water to boil.

- Once boiling, add rice and continue boiling
- Lower heat as necessary to prevent overflow, for 55 minutes.
- Remove, drain any excess water, return the rice to pot.
- Cover, let rest for 10 minutes, then stir in ¼ teaspoon of the salt.
- Place the cubed sweet potato on the pan.
- Drizzle with the olive oil and sprinkle with ¼ teaspoon of the salt. Toss to coat in oil.
- Arrange the sweet potatoes in a single layer, roast for 30 minutes in the preheated oven, tossing halfway, until tender.
- Combine extra virgin olive oil, apple cider vinegar, Dijon mustard, maple syrup, ginger, sea salt, and black pepper in a small bowl and whisk until combined. Set aside.
- Combine the arugula with wild rice and roasted sweet potatoes in a large serving bowl.
- Spread the seeds on your parchment-covered baking sheet.
- Bake for 4 minutes, until lightly golden.

- Spread the toasted seeds.
- Top with the crumbled feta, green onion, and dried cranberries.
- Serve and enjoy.

Pomegranate and pear salad with ginger dressing

Ginger is the main flavor in the pomegranate and pear salad recipe. It features vegetables and herbs for a perfect Mediterranean Sea diet.

Ingredients

- 1 tablespoon of maple syrup
- ½ cup of raw pecans
- 5 ounces of baby arugula
- 1 tablespoon of apple cider vinegar
- ¼ teaspoon of fine sea salt
- 10 twists of freshly ground black pepper
- 2 ounces of goat cheese
- 1 tablespoon of Dijon mustard
- 1 large ripe Bartlett pear
- 1 honey crisp
- 1 teaspoon of finely grated fresh ginger
- Arils from 1 pomegranate
- ¼ cup of extra virgin olive oil

Directions

- Place the pecans in a skillet over medium heat.

- Toast, stirring often, until fragrant for 5 minutes or so.
- Remove, and roughly chop. Set aside.
- Arrange the arugula across a large serving platter.
- Sprinkle the chopped pecans and crumbled goat cheese over the arugula.
- Arrange slices of pear and apple across the salad in sections.
- Then, sprinkle all over with fresh pomegranate arils.
- Combine extra virgin olive oil, apple cider vinegar, Dijon mustard, maple syrup, ginger, sea salt, and black pepper, whisk until blended.
- Taste, and adjust the seasoning.
- Drizzle the ginger dressing lightly all over the salad.
- Serve and enjoy.

Wild rice and kale salad

Ingredients

- 1 cup of cherry tomatoes
- 5 green onions
- 1 cup of wild rice
- 1 ¼ cups of water
- 2 tablespoons of extra virgin olive oil
- 1 medium red bell pepper
- 1 small of bunch kale
- ½ cup of crumbled feta cheese
- ¼ cup of lemon juice
- 1 clove garlic, pressed
- ½ teaspoon of fine sea salt
- ¼ teaspoon of ground black pepper
- 2 teaspoons of maple syrup

Directions

- Add the wild rice and water to an Instant Pot.
- Secure the lid and move the steam release valve to Sealing.
- Cook on high pressure for 22 minutes.

- Whisk together the olive oil, lemon juice, garlic, salt, pepper, and maple syrup for the dressing. Set aside.
- Add chopped kale, green onions, red bell pepper, and tomatoes to the bowl.
- Toss the vegetables to coat.
- When the cooking cycle is complete, let the pressure naturally release for 10 minutes, then move the steam release valve to Venting to release any remaining pressure.
- When the floating valve drops, remove the lid and give the rice a stir.
- Add the rice to the bowl of dressed vegetables.
- Taste and adjust the seasoning.
- Serve and enjoy.

Fresh mint dressing

Mint is as fresh as it feels in the mouth. This delicious mint dressing recipe features lemon juice and natural honey for better taste that suits a Mediterranean style.

Ingredients

- 2 cloves garlic, roughly chopped
- ½ cup of extra virgin olive oil
- ¼ teaspoon of sea salt
- ½ cup of lemon juice
- ¼ cup of packed fresh mint leaves
- 10 twists of freshly ground black pepper
- 3 tablespoons of honey
- 1 tablespoon of Dijon mustard

Directions

- In a food processor, combine all of the above ingredients and blend until smooth.
- Taste, and adjust the seasoning accordingly.
- Serve and enjoy.
- Any leftover should be refrigerated for up to 1 week.

155. Fattoush salad with mint dressing

Ingredients

- ½ cup of chopped radish
- 2 whole grain pitas
- ½ cup of torn fresh mint leaves
- 2 tablespoons of extra virgin olive oil
- ½ cup of crumbled feta
- 1 cup of chopped red onion
- Pinch of fine sea salt
- ½ batch of fresh mint dressing
- Ground sumac
- 10 ounces of fresh romaine lettuce
- 1 large tomato, chopped
- 1 cup of quartered and thinly sliced Persian cucumber

Directions

- Preheat your oven to 400°F.
- Toss the torn pita with 2 tablespoons olive oil until lightly coated.
- Sprinkle with salt, bake in the oven until the pieces golden in 12 minutes, tossing halfway.
- Let to cool.

- In a large serving bowl, combine the chopped lettuce together with the tomatoes, cucumber, parsley, onion, radish, mint, and feta, and toasted pita.
- Drizzle with ½ cup of the dressing over the salad.
- Gently toss to lightly coated in dressing.
- Serve and enjoy sprinkled with sumac.

Fresh herbed avocado salad

Ingredients

Variety of herb mix is used to cover the avocado with lime honey dressing and toasted pepitas. It is as healthy as any other Mediterranean Sea diet recipe.

Ingredients

- 2 teaspoons honey or maple syrup
- ½ cup raw pepitas
- Extra virgin olive oil
- ¼ teaspoon chili powder
- ½ teaspoon fine sea salt
- Pinch of salt
- ½ chopped radish
- ½ cup chopped green onion
- ¼ cup lime juice
- Lime zest for garnish
- ½ cup chopped fresh cilantro, parsley, basil, dill
- 1 medium jalapeño
- 4 large just-ripe avocados

Directions

- Toast the pepitas in a large skillet over medium heat, stirring often, until golden on the edges.
- Remove, stir in the chili powder together with the olive oil and pinch of salt. Let cool.
- In a mixing dish, combine the chopped radish, green onion, herbs and jalapeño. Set aside.
- Then, whisk together the lime juice, olive oil, honey, and salt in a small bowl. Set aside.
- Place the avocado in a medium serving bowl.
- Drizzle the dressing all over it.
- Stir the toasted pepitas into the herb mix, then spoon it over the avocados.
- Serve and enjoy.

Sliced fennel, orange and almond salad

Ingredients

- Sherry vinegar
- 3 bulbs of fennel
- Extra virgin olive oil
- 1 handful of almonds
- 2 handfuls of rocket
- 3 oranges
- A few springs of fresh mint

Directions

- Peeler and place the fennel in a bowl of ice water.
- Toast the almonds in a dry frying pan, crush in a pestle.
- Arranged slice the oranges on a platter.
- Drain the fennel, mix together with the mint, rocket, a splash of sherry vinegar and oil.
- Season with sea salt and black pepper
- Scatter the fennel mixture over the oranges topping with toasted almonds.
- Serve and enjoy.

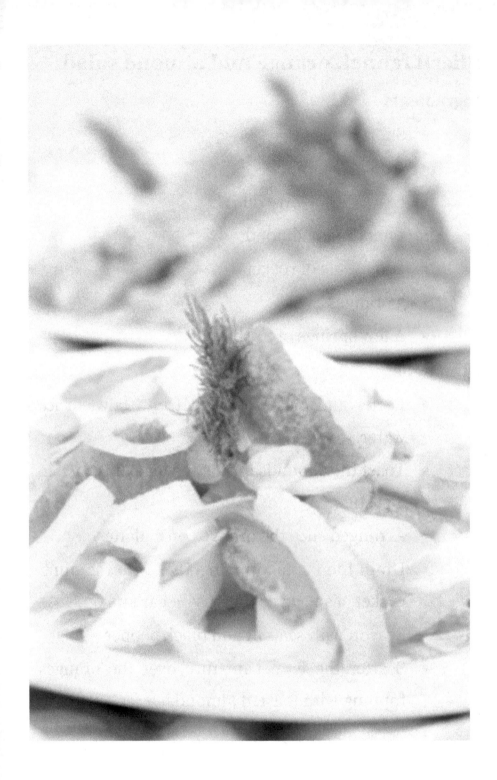

Roasted squash and couscous salad

Ingredients

- 2 tablespoons of pumpkin seeds
- 1 butternut squash
- 1 fresh green chili
- ½ of a lemon
- 5 sprigs of fresh thyme
- 100g of couscous
- 1 tablespoon cumin seeds
- Olive oil

Directions

- Preheat the oven to 375°F.
- Place the squash and chili into a roasting dish.
- Spread over the cumin seeds together with thyme sprigs, and olive oil.
- Season with sea salt.
- Let roast for 50 minutes, or until lightly golden, turning halfway.
- Place the couscous in a bowl, add enough boiling water above the couscous.
- Cover the bowl and leave for 10 minutes.

- Toast the pumpkin seeds in a dry frying pan.
- Stir in the lemon zest and juice, roasted squash and olive oil.
- Serve and enjoy wit scattered pumpkin seeds.

Spicy cucumber pickle

Ingredients

- 150ml of vinegar
- 2 banana shallots
- 2-star anise
- 2 teaspoons of mustard seeds
- 6 pickling cucumbers
- ½ teaspoon of ground turmeric
- 75g of caster sugar

Directions

- Place the cucumbers together with the shallots in a colander.
- Sprinkle with 2 teaspoons of sea salt.
- Rinse after 45 minutes.
- Combine all the other ingredients in a pan let boil.
- Stir until the sugar dissolves.
- Fit the cucumbers snugly into a jar.
- Pour over the liquid.
- Seal and leave for 24 hours.
- Serve and enjoy.

Spicy feta and pepper dip

Ingredients

- 3 tablespoons of olive oil
- 240g of feta cheese
- 120g of jarred red peppers

Directions

- Combine the feta, olive oil, and red pepper in a blender.
- Season with black pepper, then blend until smooth.
- Transfer to a serving bowl.
- Serve and enjoy.

Brazilian fish stew (Moqueca)

This incredible Mediterranean fish stew features coconut milk with lime and jalapeno with favorite flavors perfect for any meal.

Ingredients

- 1 teaspoon of salt
- ½ cup chopped cilantro, scallions
- 1 lime- zest and juice
- 3 tablespoons of coconut
- 1 14 ounce can of coconut milk
- 1 cup of fish or chicken stock
- 1 onion- finely diced
- 1 pounds of firm white fish- Halibut
- 2 teaspoons of paprika
- 1 cup of carrot, diced
- 1 red bell pepper, diced
- Squeeze of lime
- 4 garlic cloves- rough chopped
- ½ jalapeno, finely diced
- 1 tablespoon of tomato paste
- 1 teaspoon of ground cumin

- 1 cups of tomatoes, diced

Directions

- Place pat dry fish cut in pieces in a bowl.
- Add salt together with the zest from half the lime and lime juice massage to coat. Set aside.
- In a large pan, heat the olive oil over medium heat.
- Then, add onion together with salt , let sauté 3 minutes.
- Lower the heat, add carrot with bell pepper, garlic, and jalapeno.
- Allow to cook for 5 minutes.
- Add tomato paste with the spices and stock.
- Mix and let simmer, then add tomatoes.
- Cover, continue to simmer over low heat for 5 minutes.
- Add the coconut milk and season accordingly.
- Nestle the fish in the stew and simmer until cooked through in6 minutes.
- Spoon the flavorful coconut broth over the fish cook until desired.
- Taste and adjust accordingly.

- Serve and enjoy with rice.

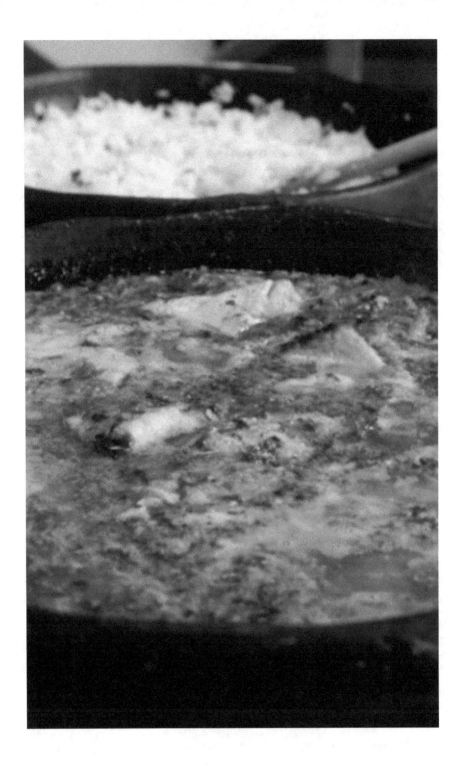

Simple salmon chowder

Ingredients

- 1/3 cup of vermouth
- 3 tablespoons of olive oil
- Fennel fronds, lemon wedges, fresh dill
- 1 onion, diced
- 3 cups of fish or chicken stock
- 1 teaspoon of salt
- 1 small fennel bulb,
- 1 lb. salmon, skinless
- 1 cup of celery, sliced
- 2 cups of whole milk
- 4 garlic cloves, rough chopped
- 1 teaspoon of fennel seeds
- ½ teaspoon of thyme
- ½ teaspoon of smoked paprika
- ¾ lb. of baby potatoes, thinly sliced
- 1 bay leaf

Directions

- Start by heating olive oil over medium heat.

- Sauté the onion with fennel and celery for 6 minutes.
- Add garlic with fennel seeds , thyme, and sauté again briefly, stirring.
- Add the smoked paprika .
- Add vermouth let cook for 2 minutes.
- Then, add the stock together with the salt , thyme and bay, simmer over high heat.
- Add potatoes and stir.
- Cover, bring to a simmer over low heat until tender in 10 minutes
- Add the milk and bring to a low simmer.
- Add the salmon, poach in the soup for 2 minutes.
- Taste, and adjust seasonings accordingly.
- Serve and enjoy garnished with fennel fronds, lemon wedges, and or fresh dill.

Furikake salmon bowls

This furikake salmon bowls are a delicious Mediterranean Sea diet fish recipe elevated by the shiitake mushrooms, avocado, and cabbage

Ingredients

- 2 extra-large handfuls of shredded cabbage
- 10 ounces of salmon
- 4 ounces of shiitake mushrooms
- Scallions, furikake , cucumber, chili flakes
- 3 tablespoons of soy sauce
- 3 tablespoons of Mirin
- 2 tablespoons of sesame oil
- 1 tablespoon of Furikake
- 2 cups of cooked rice
- Pinch of salt , pepper and chili flakes
- 1 avocado , sliced

Directions

- Cook rice according to the package Directions.
- Mix soy sauce together with the mirin in a small bowl.

- Then, heat the sesame oil in a large skillet over medium high heat.
- Season with a pinch of salt , pepper and chili flakes.
- Add the salmon with mushrooms, and sear all sides, until turns golden.
- Turn off the heat let cool slightly.
- Spoon sauce over top of the salmon and mushrooms, swirling the skillet. Keep aside for later.
- Divide rice between 2 bowls.
- Sprinkle with furikake .
- Organize the cabbage and avocado wedges in the bowl.
- Top with seared salmon and mushrooms.
- Sprinkle with Furikake and the remaining sauce over the avocado and cabbage.
- Serve and enjoy immediately.

Lemony zucchini noodles with halibut

Ingredients

- 16 ounces of zucchini noodles
- 1 garlic clove, smashed
- Sweet cherry tomatoes, chili flakes, optional
- 2 tablespoons of olive oil
- 2 teaspoons lemon zest
- Salt and pepper to taste
- ½ cup chopped Italian parsley
- 10 ounces of halibut
- 1 tablespoon of olive oil
- 1 fat shallot, sliced thin
- 3 garlic cloves, rough chopped
- 1 tablespoon lemon juice

Directions

- Preheat your oven ready to 375F.
- Heat oil in a medium skillet over medium heat.
- When hot enough, add smashed garlic clove and swirl to infuse.
- Pat fish dry and season with salt and pepper searing both sides until golden.

- Place in the warm oven until cooked through in 6 minutes.
- In a large skillet, heat another oil over medium heat.
- Add shallots together with the garlic, stirring until fragrant in 3 minutes.
- Then, add the zucchini noodles, season with salt and pepper.
- Sauté until noodles for 4 minutes.
- Toss in lemon zest, fresh parsley, and a squeeze of lemon.
- Taste, and adjust accordingly.
- Divide among two bowls and top with the halibut.
- Serve and enjoy.

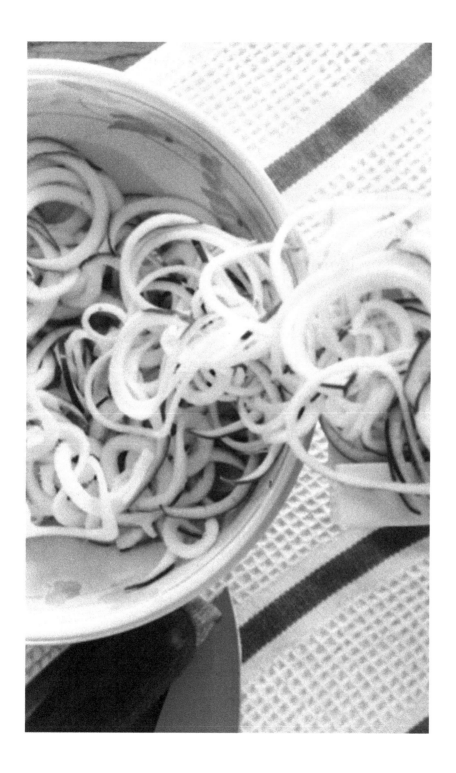

Spicy miso ramen with chili roasted salmon and bok choy

This recipe is perfect for a vegan and Mediterranean Sea diet. It draws it distinction from the mushrooms, scallions, roasted chili and paleo.

Ingredients

- 3 scallions
- 6 ounces of salmon, thinly sliced
- 4 ounces of shitake mushrooms
- 4 ounces of fresh ramen noodles
- 2 tablespoons of soy sauce
- 2 baby bok choy – sliced, lengthwise
- 2 teaspoons of honey or maple
- 3 teaspoons of garlic chili paste
- 4 cups of chicken broth
- 2 tablespoons of miso paste
- ½ teaspoon of hondashi granules
- 1 tablespoon of toasted sesame oil

Directions

- Preheat your oven ready to 400 F.

- Stir the soy sauce together with the honey , sesame oil , and chili paste in a small bowl.
- Brush the marinade over both sides of salmon and shitakes.
- Place on a parchment lined baking sheet.
- Let broil for 5 minutes, set aside.
- Bring the stock to a simmer in a medium pot .
- Add miso with hondashi, stir until combined.
- Add the bok choy and scallions, let wilt.
- Lower heat let simmer.
- Taste, and adjust seasoning accordingly.
- Divide the noodles among two bowls.
- Top with the salmon and shitakes.
- Organize the bok choy around the noodles, ladling the flavorful broth on top.
- Garnish with fresh scallions or crispy shallots
- Serve and enjoy.

Wood-fired shellfish

Ingredients

- Extra virgin olive oil
- 2 kg of mixed seafood
- 2 lemons
- Freshly ground black pepper
- 2 cloves garlic, peeled
- A few sprigs of soft fresh herbs
- Sea salt

Ingredients

- Start by firing up your wood-fired oven ready to 380°F.
- Clean and wash the shellfish, pulling the beards off the mussels, discard any open ones.
- Bash the garlic with a good pinch of sea salt in a pestle and mortar until creamy, then grate in the lemon zest.
- Add a good pinch of black pepper with enough extra virgin olive oil to make a dressing.
- Place the shellfish into a large roasting tray.
- Drizzle with the dressing, toss together.

- Spread the shellfish out into an even layer.
- Add halved lemon to the tray, slide into the hot oven, roast for 10 minutes.
- Serve and enjoy with herb leaves.

Smoky barbecue shellfish

Ingredients

- 2kg of shellfish
- 2 handfuls of fresh flat-leaf parsley
- 1 clove of garlic
- Herb branches
- 3 lemons
- 4 fresh red chilies
- Extra virgin olive oil

Directions

- Begin by adding the garlic together with the lemon zest and juice to a large bowl.
- Pour in 3 times the amount of extra virgin olive oil with finely chopped parsley stalks. Mix.
- Smoke the herb branches on the Barbie.
- Drain the shellfish, throw onto the hottest part of the Barbie.
- Lift the sides up after 3 minutes to check the shellfish have opened.
- Remove them to the dressing bowl, remove out any shellfish that have not opened.

- Sprinkle over many chopped parsley and chili, mix together.
- Serve and enjoy.

Garlic prawn kebabs

Ingredients

- 20g feta cheese
- Olive oil
- 75g of sourdough bread
- Extra virgin olive oil
- 1 lemon
- 160g of raw peeled king prawns
- 1 x 400g tin of cherry tomatoes
- ½ x 460g jar of roasted red peppers
- 3 cloves of garlic
- ½ a bunch of flat-leaf parsley

Directions

- Preheat the grill to high.
- Slice and cut the bread into 3cm chunks, place in a large bowl with the prawns, sliced peppers, garlic, parsley, half of lemon juice, olive oil, a pinch of black pepper, and stalk. Mix well.
- Skewer up the prawns and bread on 2 skewers, interlacing with the peppers.

- Sit each skewer across a roasting tray, grilling for 8 minutes, turning halfway.
- Place a non-stick frying pan on a medium heat.
- Add ½ a tablespoon of olive oil and the sliced garlic, stir regularly for 2 minutes.
- Pour in the tinned tomatoes to bubble away until the skewers are ready.
- Add a squeeze of lemon juice, then season the sauce to taste.
- Serve the kebabs on top of the sauce, sprinkled with feta and black pepper.
- Serve and enjoy with extra virgin olive oil.

Grilled Scottish langoustines

Ingredients

- 40g of unsalted butter
- 10 medium langoustines
- 1 lemon
- 25g of 'nduja

Directions

- Add 40g sea salt to 2 liters of water, bring to a boil in a large pan.
- Have a large bowl ready with 2 liters of ice-cold water.
- Plunge the langoustines into the boiling water briefly, remove and refresh in the cold water, let dry.
- Preheat the grill to medium high heat.
- In a blender, process the 'nduja with 20ml of warm water until smooth.
- Add the butter, blend to combine.
- Lay the langoustines cut-side-up on a large roasting tray, loosen them within their shells, and spoon over the 'nduja butter.

- Transfer Place under the grill until the butter is bubbling and the langoustines are golden.
- Finish with a squeeze of lemon juice.
- Serve and enjoy.

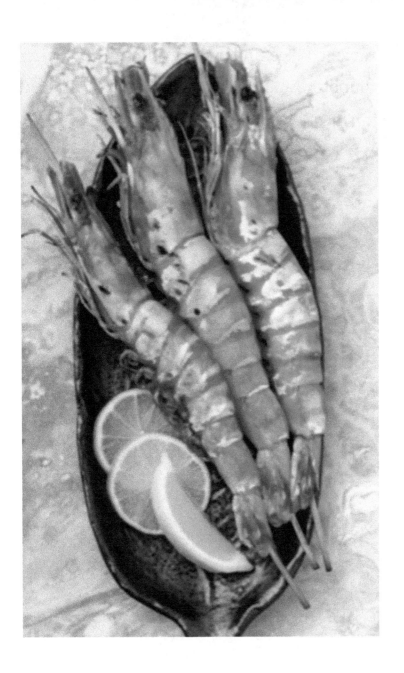

Baked clams with roasted sweet shallots and fennel

Ingredients

- 300ml of Italian white wine
- 1 large bulb of fennel
- 1 lemon
- 1 bunch of fresh flat-leaf parsley
- 1 teaspoon of fennel seeds
- 20 round shallots
- 1 teaspoon of dried chili flakes
- Olive oil
- 1.8kg of large Italian clams

Directions

- Preheat the oven to 350°F.
- Place the shallots with cut-side-up in a large roasting tray.
- Add fennel wedges to the tray.
- Bash fennel seeds with chili flakes in a pestle and mortar, then sprinkle over the shallots.
- Drizzle over 4 tablespoons of olive oil, season.

- Let bake in the oven for 25 minutes, or until the shallots are golden.
- Remove the shallots and fennel from the oven.
- Raise the heat to the maximum.
- Add the clams to the tray of juices and pour over the wine.
- Pick and finely chop the parsley, grate the lemon zest, mix most of it through.
- Rub the halved lemon with olive oil, then place in the pan, then cover the dish with tin foil.
- Let bake for 15 minutes.
- Sprinkle the remaining lemon zest and parsley over the dish and gently fold everything through the cooking juices.
- Serve and enjoy with chilled Italian wine and crusty bread.

Sizzling seared scallops

Ingredients

- 8 raw king scallops
- 200g of frozen peas
- 50g of firm black pudding
- 400g of potatoes
- ½ a bunch of fresh mint

Directions

- Cook chopped potatoes in a pan of boiling salted water for 12 minutes.
- Add the peas for the last 3 minutes.
- Place a non-stick frying pan on a medium high heat.
- Place 1 tablespoon of olive oil once hot, with the remaining mint leaves in to crisp briefly.
- Then, scoop the leaves on to a plate, leave the olive oil in the pan.
- Season the scallops with sea salt and black pepper.
- Let fry for 2 minutes on each side, or until golden.

- Crumble in the black pudding.
- Drain the peas with the potatoes, then, return to the pan, mash with the chopped mint and 1 tablespoon of extra virgin olive oil.
- Taste, and adjust the seasoning.
- Serve and enjoy drizzled with extra virgin olive oil and sprinkle over the crispy mint.

Smoked salmon blinis

Ingredients

- 1 cup of semi-skimmed milk
- 1 cup of self-rising flour
- Unsalted butter
- 1 large egg
- Olive oil

Directions

- Place the flour with a pinch of sea salt in a large mixing bowl.
- Make a well in the center, then, crack in the egg with 1 tablespoon of olive oil, beat into the flour.
- Gently whisk in the milk until smooth batter forms.
- Put a large non-stick frying pan on a medium heat.
- Add 1 small knob of butter to melt.
- Once melted, add tablespoons of batter to the pan.
- Let, cook for 1 minute on each side, flipping over when they turn golden on the bottom.

- Transfer the cooked blinis to a plate.
- Then, continue with the remaining batter until it is all used up.
- Serve and enjoy with combos.

Potted shrimp and crab

Ingredients

- 170g of white crabmeat
- 1 lemon
- 250g of unsalted butter
- ½ a bunch of fresh dill
- 1 whole nutmeg
- 180g of brown shrimp

Directions

- Start by placing 100g of the butter into a pan over a medium heat for 10 minutes.
- Strain the liquid into a separate bowl, let cool, and discard the leftover milky liquid.
- Melt the remaining butter in a pan over a low heat, let cool briefly.
- Chop and add stalks of dill with shrimp and crab into a bowl.
- Grate half the lemon zest into the bowl, then squeeze in half the juice.
- Grate in a little nutmeg, pour in the melted butter.

- Then, season with sea salt and white pepper.
- Spoon into a serving bowl, topping with the clarified butter, and scattered with the rest of the dill.
- Refrigerate for 2 hours.
- Serve and enjoy with crunchy radishes.

Prawn cocktail

Ingredients

- 1 swig of brandy
- 100g of mixed white and brown crabmeat
- Olive oil
- ½ a clove of garlic
- Cayenne pepper
- 1 small punnet of salad cress
- 1 heaped teaspoon of ketchup
- 8 unpeeled, large, raw tiger prawns
- ¼ of an iceberg lettuce
- 4 tablespoons of mayonnaise
- 50g of brown shrimps
- ¼ of a cucumber
- 2 ripe tomatoes
- 1 sprig of fresh mint
- 50g of peeled little prawns
- Lemon

Directions

- Heat olive oil in a pan over a high heat.

- Add crushed garlic, 1 pinch of cayenne pepper, and the tiger prawns.
- Toss 4 minutes, or till cooked through.
- Remove, and set aside.
- Then, combine the lemon juice together with the remaining ingredients in a bowl, keep aside.
- Layer sliced cucumber, shredded lettuce, mint leaves, and diced tomatoes in the bowl with most of the cress.
- Add the peeled prawns, then, dollop with Marie rose sauce, finish with crabmeat, shrimps.
- Add a pinch of cayenne pepper and hang a hot prawn on the side of the bowl.
- Serve and enjoy with lemon wedges squeezed over.

Cantonese-style steamed oyster

Ingredients

- 1 tablespoon of light soy sauce
- 16 large oysters, shells intact
- 2 fresh red chilies
- 1 teaspoon of chili bean sauce
- A few sprigs of fresh coriander
- 3 spring onions
- 3 tablespoons of groundnut oil
- 5cm piece of ginger
- 2 tablespoons of dark soy sauce
- 2 cloves of garlic
- 1 tablespoon of Shaoxing rice wine

Directions

- Clean and divide the oyster between 2 heatproof plates.
- Then, set up a steamer, fill with 5cm water.
- Bring to the boil over a high heat.
- Place 1 plate of oysters in the steamer covered.
- Lower the heat, steam the oysters gently for 5 minutes.

- Combine spring onions (shredded), chopped ginger, garlic, and chili with all the other ingredients apart from oil and coriander, add in a heatproof bowl.
- Heat a large frying pan over a high heat until hot.
- Add the olive oil until slightly smoking, then pour it over the sauce.
- Remove the first batch of oysters from the steamer. stirs.
- Remove the top shells of the oysters and drizzle a bit of sauce over each one.
- Serve and enjoy with coriander leaves.

Brown shrimp on the toast

Ingredients

- 100ml of cider
- 1 knob of unsalted butter
- 4 slices of bread
- 200g of brown shrimps

Directions

- Firstly, melt the butter in a pan over medium heat.
- Then, add the shrimps.
- Pour in the cider and bring to the boil.
- Then, lower the heat, let simmer for 3 minutes, or until the cider has reduced.
- Season with pepper.
- Toast your bread, then top with the shrimps.
- Serve and enjoy.

Lobster burger

Ingredients

- 2 ripe tomatoes
- 800g of cooked lobsters
- Olive oil
- 1 heaped teaspoon of Dijon mustard
- ½ a fresh red chili
- 4 thin rashers of smoked streaky bacon
- Red wine vinegar
- 4 burger buns
- 1 clove of garlic
- 1 red onion
- Tomato ketchup
- Mayonnaise
- Extra virgin olive oil
- 1 lemon
- 1 handful of watercress
- 1 soft round lettuce

Directions

- Grate the tomatoes to a slurry on both sides, discarding the seeds and skin.

- Grate in the chili, season well.
- Then, add olive oil, a swig of vinegar, and stir in bit of fresh herbs.
- Slice the lobster after twisting off the tails.
- Leave the shell on.
- Toss the chunks in olive oil, sea salt, black pepper, and mustard.
- Let barbecue for 3 minutes on each side until cooked. Peel.
- Also, barbecue the bacon, turning frequently till golden and crispy.
- Toast the buns at the same time, then lay the bottom halves on a nice board.
- Rub garlic over each side of halved buns.
- Drizzle with oil, then add a tiny blob of ketchup, with bit of mayo and a squeeze of lemon juice.
- Place the lettuce leaves, one onto each bun with a wodge of watercress.
- Top with the lobster and salsa, then, crumble over the bacon.

- Scatter over some sliced red onion, topping with the bun lid.
- Secure the burgers with skewers.
- Serve and enjoy.

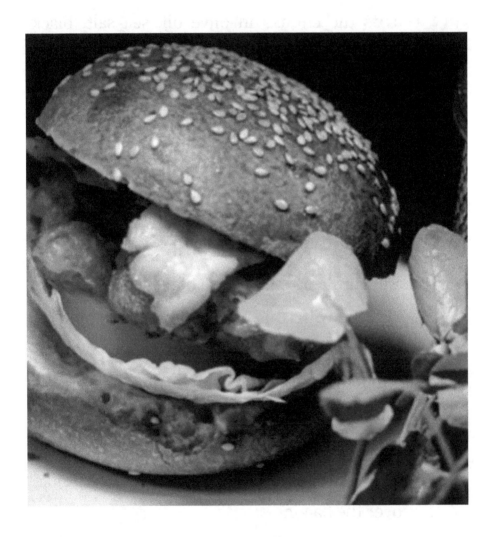

Grilled lobster rolls

Ingredients

- 2 tablespoons of mayonnaise
- 85g of butter
- 6 submarine rolls
- 1 stick of celery
- ½ of an iceberg lettuce
- 500g of cooked lobster meat

Directions

- Preheat a griddle pan until really hot.
- Butter the rolls on both sides and grill until toasted on both sides and lightly charred.
- Combine the celery, chopped lobster meat with the mayonnaise.
- Season with sea salt and black pepper to taste.
- Open warm grilled buns, shred and pile the lettuce inside each one.
- Then, top with the lobster mixture.
- Serve and enjoy right away.

Charred prawns in sweet aubergine sauce

Ingredients

- 2 aubergines
- 4 cloves of garlic
- Olive oil
- 2 large bunches of fresh basil
- 1kg of ripe tomatoes
- 1 teaspoon of dried oregano
- 2 fresh red chilies
- 3 tablespoons of red wine vinegar
- 16 king prawns

Directions

- Combine garlic, basil leaves, chilies, red wine vinegar, olive oil, and seasoning in a blender, process to a paste.
- Remove the prawn shells, then, cut along the back of each, and open up like a book.
- Place into a bowl with basil paste, mix to coat.
- Cover the bowl with Clingfilm, let marinate in the fridge for overnight.

- Score a cross in the top of each tomato, place in a large bowl and cover with boiling water.
- Drain the tomatoes, peel the skins, chop the flesh. Set aside.
- Place a saucepan over a medium heat, add olive oil.
- Add aubergines and fry for 10 minutes, stirring frequently.
- Add the remaining chili, garlic, oregano, and basil stalk into the pan, fry briefly, stir in the tomatoes.
- Add a few splashes of water, let simmer over low heat for about 30 minutes.
- Place a griddle pan over a high heat.
- Once hot enough, cook the prawns for 2 minutes on each side.
- Drop the prawns into the sauce.
- Stir the remaining basil leaves into the sauce.
- Serve and enjoy.

Spicy prawn curry with quick Pilau rice

Ingredients

- 1 teaspoon of cumin seeds
- 1 small red onion
- 1 teaspoon of unsalted butter
- ½ a bunch of fresh coriander
- 5cm piece of ginger
- 1 onion
- 1 fresh green chili
- ½ mug of basmati rice
- olive oil
- 1 teaspoon of mustard seeds
- vegetable oil
- Turmeric
- 2 ripe tomatoes
- 200g of raw king prawns, shells on
- 1 fresh bay leaf
- 100ml of light coconut milk
- 3 cardamom pods
- 4 cloves

Directions

- Heat 1 tablespoon of olive oil over a medium heat.
- Add the red onion together with the coriander stalks, and dried spices, then fry for 1 minute.
- Add the chopped ginger with the green chili, then cook for a further 5 minutes, stirring occasionally.
- Add onion with vegetable oil and butter to a pan over a medium heat.
- Let cook for 5 minutes, then, place a kettle of water on to boil.
- Sprinkle in the spices, let cook for 1 minute.
- Raise the heat, then, add the rice, stir well, add water twice the size of the rice mug, cook over reduced heat with a pinch of salt.
- Simmer for 15 minutes over a low heat, or until the water has been absorbed.
- Add the fresh tomatoes to the spiced onions with a splash of boiling water.
- Bring to the boil, season, then simmer for 5 minutes.

- Stir in the prawns together with the coconut milk, let cook for 5 minutes.
- Fluff, serve and enjoy with the curry and scattering the coriander leaves on top.

Clams casino

Ingredients

- 1 knob of unsalted butter
- 10 large cherrystone clams
- 1 lemon
- 4 large cloves of garlic
- 200g of fresh white breadcrumbs
- ½ a bunch of fresh thyme
- Extra virgin olive oil
- 4 jarred red peppers
- 8 rashers of smoked streaky bacon

Directions

- Preheat the grill to high.
- Place a deep pan over a high heat.
- Add the clams with a splash of water, cover.
- Let cook over a high heat, shaking now and then, until all the clams have opened, let cool on a tray.
- Snip each bacon rasher into 3, place the pieces in a non-stick frying pan.

- Cook over a medium heat until the bacon is just starting to crisp.
- Lift the pieces of bacon out of the pan onto a plate, return the pan to the heat.
- Add the butter together with the garlic and thyme, then add the breadcrumbs when sizzling.
- Let fry for 3 minutes, stirring.
- Season with sea salt and black pepper. Remove, let cool.
- Remove the clams from the shells, chop into quarters.
- Place into a bowl, then add a squeeze of lemon juice, a drizzle of extra virgin olive oil, and a pinch of seasoning.
- Rinse the shells, spread out on a large roasting tray.
- Place a few pepper strips into each shell, then, bit of breadcrumbs.
- Nestle a couple of clam quarters in each one and cover with more crumbs.

- Top with a piece of bacon and drizzle extra virgin olive oil.
- Place the tray on a low shelf under the hot grill for 5 minutes.
- Serve and enjoy with the remaining lemon wedges squeezed over.

Boiled prawn wontons with chili dressing

Ingredients

- 20ml of light soy sauce
- 225g of raw prawns
- 1 teaspoon of dried chili flakes
- 1 spring onion
- 40ml of vegetable oil
- 1cm piece of ginger
- 20ml of rice wine vinegar
- 1 tablespoon of Sichuan pepper
- 3 tablespoons of sea salt
- 1½ teaspoon of Shaoxing wine
- 3 tablespoons light soy sauce
- White sugar
- ½ teaspoon of sesame oil
- 24 fresh wonton wrappers

Directions

- Dry-roast the Sichuan pepper with 3 teaspoons of sea salt in a heavy.
- Once popping, remove, let cool.
- Then, grind to a powder in a pestle and mortar.

- Place chili flakes in a heatproof bowl.
- Heat olive oil in a small heavy-based frying pan until it shimmering, pour the oil over the chili to release the flavor.
- Stir, then let stand, uncovered, for 30 minutes.
- Sieve the oil over a bowl, then, mix with remaining dressing ingredients.
- Place the prawn meat, spring onion, ginger, and the remaining ingredients except for wonton, in a bowl.
- Place in the refrigerator for 30 minutes covered.
- Place a rounded teaspoon of prawn filling in the center of a wrapper.
- Dip your finger in some water and moisten the bottom edge of the wrapper, then fold it in half.
- Hold the wonton lengthways with the folded edge down.
- Fold in half lengthways, then lightly moisten one corner of the folded edge.

- Bring the two ends together with a twisting action, and seal.
- Bring a large pan of water to the boil.
- Then, drop the wontons, in batches, into the water, let cook for 2 minutes.
- Serve and enjoy with the dressing, and sprinkled with Sichuan seasoning, prepared at the beginning.

Prawn and crab wontons

Ingredients

- 200g of white crabmeat
- 30 wonton wrappers
- 1 fresh red chili
- 2 tablespoons of oyster sauce
- 200g of peeled raw tiger prawns
- Groundnut oil
- Sweet chili sauce
- ½ tablespoon of sesame oil
- Corn flour
- 1 ginger
- 1 clove of garlic
- ½ bunch of chives

Directions

- Combine ginger together with the garlic, chili, sliced chives, crabmeat, oyster sauce, sesame oil, and the prawn in a bowl. Mix to combine.
- Lay the wonton wrappers on a clean work surface, cover with a damp.
- Lightly dust a tray with corn flour.

- Spoon 1 teaspoon of the filling onto the middle of a wrapper.
- Brush the edges with a little water, then bring up over the filling, seal.
- Place on the flour-dusted tray, then repeat with the remaining ingredients.
- Pour boiling water into a saucepan over a medium-high heat.
- Bring to the boil.
- Cut out a circle of greaseproof paper so it fits snugly into a bamboo steamer, grease one side with oil, then place oil-side up into the steamer.
- Add the wontons in a single layer, then place the basket on top of the pan, steam for 8 minutes covered.
- Serve and enjoy with chili sauce.

Langoustines with lemon and pepper butter

Ingredients

- 100g of butter
- 1kg of fresh langoustines
- 2 teaspoons of coarse black pepper
- Olive oil
- 400 ml white wine
- 50g of fresh breadcrumbs
- 1 lemon
- 2 lemons

Directions

- Combine the lemon zest, butter, black pepper, and a pinch of salt, keep for later.
- Heat a grill to high.
- Combine the langoustines and wine in a pan.
- Bring to the boil, then lower the heat, let simmer for 5 minutes covered.
- Place your langoustines, belly-side down, on a chopping board, cut in half lengthways, discarding the black vein in the tail.

- Place, flesh-side up, on a baking tray, topping with the lemon butter, sprinkle over the breadcrumbs and drizzle with oil.
- Grate the zest from 1 lemon into a bowl.
- Place the lemon halves on the tray.
- Let grill for 10 minutes.
- Serve and enjoy sprinkled with zest and grilled lemon.

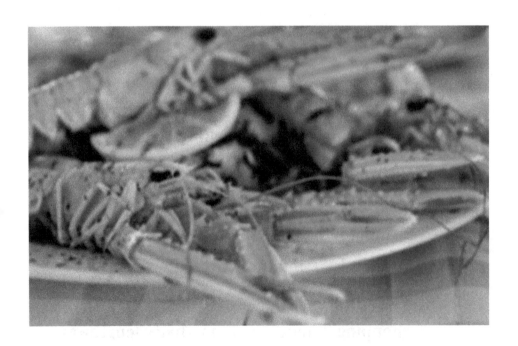

Szechuan sweet and sour prawns

Ingredients

- 150ml of unsweetened pineapple juice
- 300g of pineapple
- 1 tablespoon of low-salt soy sauce
- 1 red pepper
- 1 yellow pepper
- ½ bunch of fresh coriander
- 3 tablespoons of rice vinegar
- 2 cloves of garlic
- 2 fresh red chilies
- Sea salt
- 1 ginger
- ½ tablespoon of corn flour
- 24 peeled raw king prawns
- Groundnut oil

Directions

- Preheat a large griddle pan over a high heat.
- Add the pineapple for 4 minutes, turning occasionally.
- Remove, let cool on a board.

- Add sliced peppers to the griddle for about 3 minutes, turning halfway.
- Bash the garlic together with the chilies, and a pinch of salt to a rough paste, in a pestle and mortar.
- Add the ginger, then bash until broken down, combined.
- Place the chili paste into a large bowl with the prawns and a splash of oil, mix.
- Heat a lug of oil in a large non-stick frying pan over a medium-high heat.
- Add the prawn mixture, let fry for 4 minutes.
- Then, chop the cooled pineapple into bite-sized chunks.
- In a bowl, combine the pineapple juice together with the vinegar, soy, corn flour, and a splash of water, add to the pan along with the chargrilled pineapple and peppers.
- Bring to the boil, then, simmer over a low heat for about 2 minutes
- Serve and enjoy with steamed rice.

Cooked oyster with burnt butter

Ingredients

- ½ of a lemon
- 800g of rock salt
- 40g of unsalted butter
- 8 rock oysters
- Tabasco sauce

Directions

- Preheat the oven to the maximum heat.
- Place the rock salt into an ovenproof frying pan.
- Place the rock salt in the oven to preheat for around 20 minutes.
- Then, place in the oysters on top, return the pan to the oven for 10 minutes.
- Melt the butter in a frying pan over a medium heat, then cook for 3 minutes, or until the oyster turns to deep golden.
- Add a few drops of Tabasco to taste.
- Remove from heat, add a squeeze of lemon juice, swirling the pan until combined.

- Put the pan to one side.
- Insert an oyster knife in, then carefully lever it open.
- Discard the oyster tops, then place the bottom shells with the oyster on a platter.
- Serve and enjoy with a drizzle over the burnt butter.

Cajun blackened fish steaks

Ingredients

- 2 level teaspoons of smoked paprika
- 4 x 200g of white fish fillets
- 1 teaspoon of cayenne pepper
- Lemon
- 10 sprigs of fresh thyme
- 2 tablespoons of olive oil
- 4 sprigs of fresh oregano
- 2 cloves of garlic

Directions

- Bash the fresh herbs together with the garlic in a pestle and mortar until coarse paste forms.
- Then, mix in the spices with bit of sea salt, black pepper, olive oil, and a squeeze of the juice of half the lemon, stir well.
- Lightly score the skin of your fish in lines about 2cm apart.
- Smear the rub all over both sides of the fish.
- Place a pan over a medium-high heat.

- Place the fish in the pan, skin side down, let cook for 4 minutes.
- It will get quite smoky, so you might want to open a window.
- Lower the heat, then, flip your fish over, and continue to cook for 4 minutes on the other side.
- Cut the remaining lemon half and the second lemon into wedges.
- Serve and enjoy the fish with salad and boiled potatoes dressed in good olive oil.

Barbecued langoustines with aioli

Ingredients

- 12 langoustines
- ½ clove garlic
- 1 teaspoon of sea salt
- Lemon juice
- 1 large egg yolk
- Sprigs fennel tops
- 1 teaspoon of Dijon mustard
- 300ml of extra virgin olive oil
- Freshly ground black pepper

Directions

- To make the aioli, smash the garlic together with salt in a pestle and mortar.
- Whisk the egg yolk with the mustard in a bowl, then adding olive oils to it bit by bit, the rest.
- Add the smashed garlic with lemon juice, salt and pepper.
- Lay the langoustines flat on a chopping board, with a sharp knife, saw through their shells lengthways.

- Open them out in a butterfly style and flatten them down gently.
- Season, then cook, cut-side down, across the bars on a hot Barbie for 2 minutes, then briefly on the other side.
- Sprinkle with torn fennel tops.
- Serve and enjoy with lemony aioli.

Creamy Cornish mussels

Ingredients

- 250ml of Cornish cider
- 600g of mussels
- 1 bunch of fresh chives
- 4 cloves of garlic
- 50g of clotted cream

Directions

- Discard open mussels.
- Place a large deep pan on a high heat.
- Then, pour in 1 tablespoon of olive oil, add garlic with chives, and cider.
- Bring to a fast boil, add the mussels with the clotted cream, cover and leave for 4 minutes, shaking occasionally.
- When all the mussels have opened, they are done. Discard any closed ones.
- Taste the sauce, and adjust the seasoning with sea salt and black pepper.
- Sprinkle over the remaining chives.
- Serve and enjoy.

Pesto mussels and toast

Ingredients

- 50ml of white wine
- 70g of pesto
- 160g of fresh or frozen peas
- 2 thick slices of whole meal bread
- 500g of mussels
- 200g of baby courgettes
- 200g of ripe mixed-color cherry tomatoes
- 2 sprigs of fresh basil

Directions

- Put a large pan on a medium-high heat.
- Toast the bread as the pan heats up, turn when golden.
- Remove the toast, spread one quarter of the pesto on each slice.
- Turn on the heat under the pan to full heat.
- Place in the mussels.
- Stir in the remaining pesto, together with the courgettes, tomatoes, and peas.

- Add the wine let cover and steam for 4 minutes, shaking the pan occasionally.
- When all the mussels have opened and are soft, they are done.
- Divide the mussels, vegetables, and juices between 2 large bowls.
- Pick over the basil leaves and serve with the pesto toasts on the side.
- Enjoy.

Mussels with Guinness

Ingredients

- 1 fresh bay leaf
- ½ a bunch of fresh thyme
- 1 shallot
- 250ml of Guinness
- 2 cloves of garlic
- 2 rashers of smoked bacon
- 1kg of mussels
- 50ml of double cream
- ½ a bunch of fresh flat-leaf parsley
- 1 knob of unsalted butter

Directions

- In a pan, melt the butter and sweat the shallot with the garlic and bacon for 5 minutes.
- Add half of the herbs, together with the bay and a pinch of sea salt and black pepper.
- Then, add the mussels, then the Guinness.
- Let boil, then lower the heat, let steam for 5 minutes covered.
- Stir in the cream and remaining herbs.

- Taste, and adjust the seasoning.
- Serve and enjoy with bread.

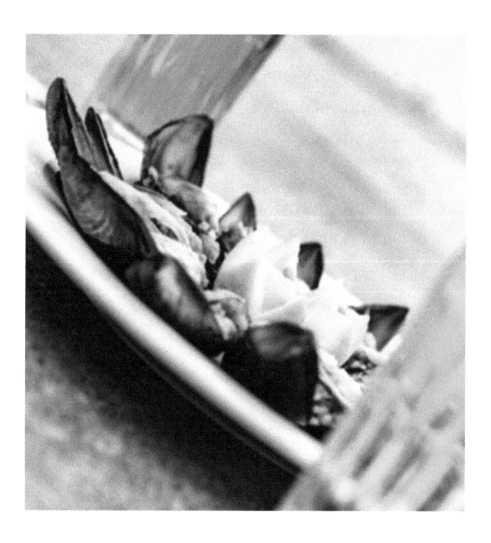

Shellfish and cider stew

Ingredients

- 1 tablespoon of unsalted butter
- 4 ripe plum tomatoes
- 3 leeks
- 600g of clams
- 600g of mussels
- 3 shallots
- 6 razor clams
- ½ a bunch of fresh flat-leaf parsley
- 500ml of organic fish stock
- 750ml of cider
- 1 teaspoon of tomato purée
- 6 langoustines
- 3 tablespoons of double cream

Directions

- Start by melting the butter in a large pan over a low heat.
- Gently fry the leeks together with the shallots, tomatoes, and parsley until soft.
- Season, then add the stock with cider.

- Raise the heat, let the liquid boil for 10 minutes, until reduces slightly.
- Warm a large serving bowl.
- Add the langoustines, cover for 3 minutes.
- Then add the razor clams. Cook for a further 2 minutes while covered.
- Add the mussels together with the clams.
- Stir gently, then, add another splash of cider, cover, let cook for a further 5 minutes, or until the mussels and clams have opened.
- Transfer the shellfish to the warmed serving bowl and put the sauce back on the heat.
- Add the cream together with the tomato purée, stir well to combine.
- Pour the sauce over the shellfish in the bowl.
- Serve and enjoy with crusty bread.

Simple baked cod with tomatoes

Simple baked cod is flavorful due to the garlic, lemon, and herbs used typically basil. It is a perfect Mediterranean Sea diet for dinner or lunch.

Ingredients

- salt, pepper and chili flakes to taste
- 3 tablespoons of olive oil
- ¼ cup of basil leaves torn
- 2 cups of cherry
- 3 garlic cloves rough chopped
- 2 lb. of cod fillets
- 1 lemon – zest and slices

Directions

- Begin by preheating your oven ready to 400°F.
- Pour the olive oil in a baking dish .
- Scatter the garlic cloves.
- Add the tomatoes with lemon slices, toss and pus to one side.
- Pat dry the fish, place in the baking dish , turn to coat each side with oil.

- Spread out the tomato garlic mixture and nestle in the fish.
- Make sure tomatoes on the sides, lemons underneath.
- Season all with salt , pepper and chili flakes.
- Let bake for 10 minutes, scatter with lemon zest.
- Continue to bake for 5 more minutes.
- Add the torn basil leaves, tossing with the warm tomatoes.
- Garnish every piece of fish with a wilted basil leaf.
- Serve and enjoy immediately.

Roasted salmon with braised lentils

Ingredients

- 7 garlic cloves, finely minced
- 1 tablespoon of fresh thyme
- 2 teaspoons of whole-grain mustard
- 2 cups of French Green Lentils
- Fresh thyme sprigs for garnish
- 2 teaspoons of lemon zest
- 2 bay leaves
- 5 sprigs of fresh thyme
- ¼ cup of sherry wine
- 3 teaspoon of salt
- pepper to taste
- 2 lbs. of salmon
- 1 onion, diced
- 1 cup of diced celery
- 5 tablespoon of olive oil
- 1 cup of diced carrot
- 4 cups of veggie

Directions

- Preheat heat oven to 325F.

- Pat dry the salmon.
- Combine garlic with thyme, whole grain, lemon zest, olive oil, salt and pepper in a small bowl.
- Brush a little marinade on the bottom sides of salmon.
- Then, place on parchment -lined sheet pan .
- Spoon the remaining over top, to form a thin layer. Set aside.
- Bake salmon in the preheated oven for 15 minutes or so.
- Heat oil in a large sauté pan over medium heat.
- Add onion together with the celery and carrots.
- Stir for 5 minutes, lower the heat, continue to cook for more 5 more minutes.
- Add the garlic and lentils.
- Cook for 2 minutes while stirring.
- Add the wine. Let this cook-off, about 2 minutes.
- Pour in the stock, salt , and mustard, and stir until combined, let simmer.

- Add the bay leaves and thyme sprigs, cover and gently simmer on low heat for 30 minutes.
- Taste and adjust accordingly.
- Serve and enjoy.

Moroccan salmon

The Moroccan salmon derives its flavor and taste from variety of fruits and vegetables and herbs. Mint and oranges are key healthy ingredients that elevate this Mediterranean Sea diet recipe.

Ingredients

- pinch of cayenne
- 2 salmon filets
- ½ teaspoon of cinnamon
- Orange zest
- ½ teaspoon of salt
- ¾ teaspoon of sugar
- 1 tablespoon of oil for searing
- ½ teaspoon of cumin

Directions

- Preheat oven to 350°F.
- In a small bowl, combine cinnamon together with the cumin, salt, sugar and cayenne.
- Sprinkle over both sides of the salmon.
- Heat oil in an oven proof skillet over medium temperature.

- Sear salmon on both sides for 2 minutes each side.
- Place in the warm oven to finish for 5 minutes.
- Garnish with orange zest.
- Serve and enjoy with Moroccan quinoa.

Pan seared salmon with chia seeds, fennel slaw and pickled onions

Ingredients

- ½ ounce of package dill
- ½ teaspoon of salt
- 3 tablespoon of lemon juice
- ¼ cup of thinly sliced sweet onion
- ½ teaspoon of dried mint, dill or tarragon
- ½ teaspoon of granulated garlic
- 1 Turkish cucumber
- 2 teaspoons of chia seeds
- Salt and pepper to taste
- 3 tablespoon of olive oil
- ½ lemon
- 2 6 ounces of wild Salmon
- 1 extra-large fennel bulb, thinly sliced

Directions

- Place fennel bulb, cucumber, dill, olive oil, lemon juice, lemon juice, salt and pepper in a medium bowl, toss well. Set aside.
- Brush the tops of salmon with olive oil .

- Place salt together with the pepper, dried herbs, granulated garlic, chia seeds in a small bowl, mix.
- Coat the top of the fish liberally with the chia mixture, pressing it down with fingers.
- Then, heat olive oil in a pan over medium heat.
- Let the pan get hot enough, then add the fish with chia seed side down and pan sear for 4 minutes until golden.
- Turnover, to keep crust intact and continue cooking until fish is cooked in 4 minutes.
- Serve and enjoy with a squeeze of lemon juice on top.

Ceviche

Ceviche is quite a delicious fish recipe that features cucumber, tomatoes, chilies, cilantro, lime and even avocado. As a result, the variety of vegetables makes this recipe a perfect Mediterranean Sea diet choice for any meal.

Ingredients

- 1 cup of diced cucumber
- ½ of a red onion, thinly sliced
- 1 pound of fresh fish- sea bass
- 1 fresh serrano chili pepper seeded
- 1 cup of grape
- 1 semi-firm avocado, diced
- 3 garlic cloves finely minced¼ teaspoon of black pepper
- ½ cup of fresh cilantro chopped
- 1 ½ teaspoon of kosher salt
- ¾ cup of fresh lime juice
- 1 tablespoon of olive oil

Directions

- Place fish together with the onion, garlic, salt , fresh chilies, pepper, and lime juice in a shallow serving bowl , mix.
- Transfer to a refrigerator to marinate for at 45 minutes.
- Gently toss in the fresh cilantro with cucumber and tomato.
- Drizzle with olive oil , mix.
- Taste, and adjust accordingly.
- Gently fold in the avocado at the end, after mixing everything.
- Serve and enjoy.

Seared Hawaiian ono with honey soy glaze and pineapple salsa

Ingredients

- 1 teaspoon of finely minced or grated ginger root
- 1 mild red chili
- 2 lbs. of Fresh Ono cut into 6 pieces
- ⅓ cup of soy sauce
- ⅓ cup of honey
- 3 teaspoon of sliced ginger
- ⅛ teaspoon of kosher salt
- 2 garlic cloves
- ¼ cup of finely diced red onion
- 1 teaspoon of olive oil
- zest and juice of one small lime
- ½ cup of chopped cilantro
- Pineapple Ginger Salsa
- ½ pineapple, pealed cored, small diced
- 1 jalapeño- seeds removed, diced

Directions

- Blend soy sauce together with the honey , garlic, sliced ginger, and olive oil in a blender until smooth.
- Put the fish and marinade in a Ziploc bag for 20 minutes or longer.
- Cut pineapple in half, saving top half for another use.
- Slice and dice into ½ inch cubes, then place in a medium bowl.
- Toss in the jalapeno, red chili, red onion, ginger root, cilantro, zest and juice and kosher salt.
- Taste, and adjust accordingly.
- Heat oil in a large heavy bottom skillet, over medium temperature.
- When oil is hot enough, place in the fish, saving the marinade.
- Sear the fish, on its sides, set aside.
- Pour the remaining marinade into the skillet let boil briefly.
- Strain and place in a small bowl.

- Spoon over the fish, with a generous amount of pineapple salsa.
- Serve and enjoy.

Sea bass with cannellini bean stew

A combination of beans and fish is an incredible protein blast. In 30 minutes, this Mediterranean Sea diet recipe will be just ready waiting for your bite.

Ingredients

- ½ teaspoon of kosher salt
- 2 tablespoons of olive oil
- ¼ teaspoon of cracked pepper
- 1 medium onion, diced
- Oil, salt and pepper for fish
- 1 cup of peeled, diced carrot
- 4 cups of chicken stock
- 1 cup of diced celery
- Italian parsley for garnish
- 4 smashed and roughly chopped garlic cloves
- 2 cups of diced tomatoes
- 4 four-ounce of sea bass fillets
- 3 cups of cannellini beans
- 1 cup of water
- 2 tablespoons of fresh sage

Directions

- In a medium heavy-bottomed pot, heat oil over medium heat.
- Add onions, stir for 2 minutes.
- Add carrots together with the celery and garlic, sauté over medium heat for 5 minutes, stirring occasionally.
- Add canned beans with the 2 cups of stock, herbs, tomatoes, salt and pepper, let boil.
- Lower the heat, cover, let simmer for 15 minutes.
- Heat 2 tablespoons of olive oil in a skillet, over medium temperature.
- Pat dry fish with paper towels.
- Season generously with kosher salt and pepper.
- Sear each side until a golden crust forms on the fish.
- Lower the heat, let cook through.
- Place the stew in a wide shallow dish topping with seared fish

- Serve and enjoy garnished with fresh Italian parsley.

CPSIA information can be obtained
at www.ICGtesting.com
Printed in the USA
LVHW081115210521
688044LV00013B/813